Embracing Your Spiritual Path

CARING
FOR A
LOVED ONE
WITH
DEMENTIA

Annie's Story

A Conversation with
PHILIP BURLEY

Also from Mastery Press:

Mastery Press

*Confronting Depression
to Stop Suicide*

The Power of Self Awareness

Love Knows No End

The Blue Island

Beyond Titanic—Voyage into Spirit

Heart's Healing

The Spirit World, Where Love Reigns Supreme

The Hum of Heaven

The Wisdom of Saint Germain

The Gift of Mediumship

Awaken the Sleeping Giant

*A Legacy of Love, Volume One:
The Return to Mount Shasta and Beyond*

To Master Self is to Master Life

A Wanderer in the Spirit Lands

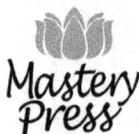

Embracing Your Spiritual Path

CARING
FOR A
LOVED ONE
WITH
DEMENTIA

Annie's Story

A Conversation with
PHILIP BURLEY

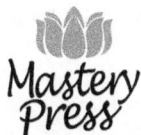

Mastery Press

Phoenix, Arizona

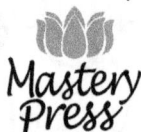

Mastery Press
P.O. Box 43548
Phoenix, AZ 85080
PB@PhilipBurley.com
(For faster service, please put
Mastery Press in the Subject line)

ISBN: 978-1-883389-22-2

Printed in the United States of America

Philip Burley portrait by Images by Kay
Scottsdale, Arizona

Cover and interior design by 1106 Design
Phoenix, Arizona

DEDICATION

This story is dedicated to people everywhere who suffer from various forms of dementia, to the vigilant caregivers who carry the burden of this disease for their loved ones as well as for themselves, and to the unsung researchers working tirelessly to identify the causes and improve the treatments for this devastating illness so that it can be eliminated from Mother Earth forever.

ACKNOWLEDGMENTS

My heartfelt appreciation goes to Annie for so honestly sharing her powerful story. Her responses to Tom's dementia reveal touching and universal human emotions surrounding loss and love and remind us all of our hidden capacity to journey on in the face of personal tragedy.

CONTENTS

Dedication 5
Acknowledgments 7
Introduction 11
A Note on Dementia 15
A New Reality 19
Staying in the Present 31
Accepting Help 37
Earthly Contraction—
    Spiritual Expansion 43
Living Well as Individuals 49
The Book of Life 55
A Different Relationship 61
Changing Needs 69
Ideas to Grow On 75
Annie's Letter 83
Afterword 87

INTRODUCTION

Are you caring for a loved one who is suffering from Alzheimer's disease or another form of dementia? If so, my conversation with Annie[1] may help you. Her husband Tom's terminal illness includes a rapidly progressive and disabling form of dementia, and she is in the process of dealing with the loss of his companionship well before his dying day. Annie is seeking to find her footing in this dire situation by understanding her own emotional needs as well as those of her husband. She also needs to know the basic medical facts of her husband's illness and increasing disability and ensure that he has the treatment and care he needs, responding to the practical and financial problems they now face.

[1] Names and some details have been changed to protect the privacy of individuals involved.

Because she has been told that this illness will end her husband's life, Annie is already grieving; but she is also highly motivated to do the best job she can in caring for him, and she desperately wants to see her situation in a universal spiritual context. Toward this end, she sought intuitive spiritual counseling with me and our conversation is the result.

Speaking with Annie was an honor because she is a genuine seeker of truth. Her intelligent search for meaning in extremely difficult circumstances is enlightening, and her articulate description of her thoughts and feelings is a gift to us all. In our conversation, Annie openly shares her inner reality, including how she is coping with her new life as a caregiver for her husband. She wants and needs to go on living, but she has been unsure of the best way to do this. How can she care for herself as well as respond to the changing needs of her husband and adult children? As you read our conversation, you will find questions and answers that may apply to you or someone you love, now or in the future.

If we believe there is nothing beyond this physical life and that death is the end, we may face our demise with despair, grief, and resignation. But Annie and I talked about a bright alternative: the prospect of an eternal journey in an afterlife where she and her husband will both be completely whole and together again.

Because of my significant and ongoing spiritual experiences since early childhood, I know that the physical body is a shell we occupy for a certain number of years before we move on to live in a higher, finer, broader, and brighter sphere in the spirit world. Once we have this understanding, life takes on new meaning, and we lose the dread of parting from someone we thought we would never see again. Instead, we look beyond the end of earthly suffering to a time when we make our own transition into the spirit world for a grand reunion with those we loved on earth.

But it is not only the hope of an eternal future that we need. By opening our hearts to grace, we can learn to experience joy and beauty differently, even amidst the most difficult circumstances. By learning to live, breathe, see, and feel in the present moment, we can touch eternity now.

May this conversation bless you with greater insight into how to live positively with chronic illness and with increased awareness that we all live in eternity from the second we are born. Yes, the body dies, but the spirit lives on. We do not die! We live forever!

—*Philip Burley*

A NOTE ON DEMENTIA

Dementia is a broad term that includes a wide range of conditions causing the loss of cognitive abilities such as language, memory, and higher reasoning. Alzheimer's disease and other specific types of dementia cause the progressive loss of cognitive abilities and critical bodily functions, leading to death unless the person dies from another condition first. The Alzheimer's Association estimates that 5.4 million Americans are affected by dementia from Alzheimer's disease.[2]

Some dementias are relatively stable if they are caused by a stroke, infection, or head injury where no progressive brain disease is present. It is

---

[2]   Alzheimer's Association. 2012 Alzheimer's disease facts and figures. *Alzheimer's and Dementia: The Journal of the Alzheimer's Association*. March 2012; 8:131–168.

reversible only when it is caused by the temporary effects of certain medications, medical conditions, or psychiatric illnesses related to depression, psychosis, or psychological or physical trauma. A neurologist can help to determine exactly what is happening to someone who exhibits signs and symptoms of dementia.

The person caring for a loved one with dementia, whatever the cause, is often over-whelmed by the degree of care needed on a 24/7 basis as well as the loss of the relationship with the ill loved one. Fear, anxiety, anger, frustration, and sadness are among the emotions the caregiver is likely to experience. Providing constant care for someone with dementia may lead to physical exhaustion and related health problems unless the caregiver receives adequate help and support.

Because of the established risk to caregivers for people with dementia and other chronic ill-nesses, a number of community services exist to provide education and support. Being with those in a similar situation can be very helpful, and support groups for caregivers are available in most localities. Respite care is usually available to relieve the primary caregiver for a number of hours daily or intermittently from individuals who come into the home or from a licensed adult day care center where care is provided in a group setting. As the condition progresses, the person with dementia may be cared for in an assisted living or skilled nursing facility, depending on the level of care needed.

Among the most valuable coping skills a caregiver can have are humor, self-awareness, and the willingness to receive help from family members, doctors, volunteers, health aides, and professionals who can provide education, information, and referrals to appropriate community resources. Maintaining positive spiritual, psychological, and philosophical perspective provides key benefits.

A NEW REALITY

Annie: Thank you for getting back to me so quickly.

Philip Burley (PB): You're very welcome. How are you?

Annie: I'm having the hardest time . . .

PB: And you know that's understandable, given the circumstances.

Annie: I guess I think I should be able to handle things better.

PB: Not necessarily. That's your thinking, but reality may be something different.

Annie: Well, that's what I'm realizing; and I'm also realizing that I need help to get to where I want to be.

PB: Well this was so unexpected. Each of us has the idea that we'll live and die a "normal" life. When and how did Tom's condition come on? And how did each of you initially respond?

Annie: I guess it began when he lost his job more than a year ago. He had a very good job, but he was given a new contract that included complicated technical tasks, and he just couldn't do it. We didn't know if the job was too hard for him or what the problem was, but they fired him because he couldn't learn the technical system needed for the new contract. He went on unemployment for a few months and looked for a simpler job. We were becoming aware that he was having more trouble with complex tasks, but we didn't think there was any big problem. He got a job as a driver but was fired three weeks later because of serious safety problems.

PB: You mean driving problems?

Annie: Yes. First, he overfilled the gas tank, and they said he damaged the vehicle and didn't report it. These kinds of mistakes were totally not who Tom is, so I knew something was very seriously wrong. He wasn't saying anything, and he didn't complain, but . . .

PB: That's his usual demeanor anyway, isn't it?

Annie: Yes. But he clearly was not driving safely, and he couldn't work on the computer anymore, so I started to think he might have experienced something like a mini-stroke and took him to a doctor.

PB: How old is he now?

Annie: He's in his early sixties. Anyway, the doctor said the tests they gave him didn't show that he'd had a stroke or anything like that. But then, over the course of about another month, he deteriorated dramatically and very rapidly. He was up all night, he became psychotic, and he thought he was dying. All he talked about was death. He was also having stomach problems. He said he was starving, the pets were starving, and the house was going to freeze in the winter. He was up all night doing obsessive things, as though he had OCD.[3] He was so scary that no one could get any sleep. I couldn't go to work and leave him at home alone.

---

[3]   Obsessive Compulsive Disorder

Finally, I went into the doctor's office with Tom and said, "I can't take it anymore. I can't go to work, he's not safe, and I don't know what's wrong with him. You have to find out!" The doctor admitted him to the hospital for a psychiatric and physical evaluation for about twelve days and did a full workup with psychiatrists, neurologists, and internists. He was ultimately diagnosed with something called "frontal temporal degeneration," and they told me his condition was terminal.

PB: Say the name of it again?

Annie: It's called "frontal temporal degeneration" or FTD, with dementia. *Frontal* refers to the frontal lobe, followed by *temporal degeneration*. They told me it affects your personality and behavior but not your memory, and he has no trouble with memory at all.

PB: Maybe that's in another area of the brain.

Annie: Right. And he has not yet developed the behavior issues they say come with this. We had a spiritual health intuitive do a reading for him, and he said Tom had about 25,000 units of mercury in his brain or some outrageous amount, so he worked on dissipating the mercury energetically.

That may have helped to prevent him from exhibiting psychotic behavior, but the doctors also put him on medications for mood stabilizing and sedation. They gave him something for trembling in his hands and something else for depression. He is on a whole set of medications.

Anyway, Tom was in the hospital for a couple weeks and then came home. They tried to get me to put him in a nursing home, and initially that's where he wanted to be, but at the last minute he decided he wanted to come home. We were very scared about that, because they said he could burn down the house. People with this condition can become very erratic and do things that are violent, even if they are completely unprovoked. Anyway, I couldn't believe it was possible that Tom would ever do anything to us. I just couldn't see it, so we risked keeping him home against the doctors' advice.

We found the day care situation for Tom about six or seven months ago, and it has worked out very well. After everything that happened before he was diagnosed, he became more his old self. He doesn't seem to be psychotic and doesn't stay up all night or talk about death all the time, but he has given up everything he loved in life.

PB: When you say he has given up everything, what you do you mean?

Annie: He has lost interest in everything. I suggested to him that he could still write stories because his life isn't over, and he could still get together with friends. He used to love photography, but I don't think he could hold a camera now. Even if he could, he's not interested. He liked science and all kinds of things, but all of those interests have stopped. He has just sort of stopped being himself.

PB: If you were to describe him today, right now, what would you say? For example, what is he doing right now?

Annie: He's at the day care center where he goes during the day. That's another thing: He seems to like being there better than he likes being at home. I think this has something to do with the fact that he is not asked to do anything that he can't do and is just taken care of at the day care. He says there's always something to do, and because they gear activities to his abilities he feels successful. His mind is very focused on himself and his needs, and not much else.

PB: Yes.

Annie: We can't carry on a meaningful conversation. He doesn't inquire about how the kids are, and he never asks me how I am. He can't relate if I tell him I had a rough day. He'll just say, "Well, when is my dinner?" It's very much not him as he was, and that's hard for me. I feel like I'm taking care of a body but not really communicating with my husband. He's more like a son than a husband at this point. I still worry that his condition could progress, and I still wonder if they really diagnosed it correctly. Maybe there is something else we could be doing . . .

PB: Have you had a second opinion? Did you see any other doctors?

Annie: Well, there were many different doctors at the hospital and different neurologists saw him.

PB: And they all concurred?

Annie: Yes. I also took him to a psychiatrist after they put him on psychiatric medications. They all agree with the diagnosis—at least that it makes sense. But he hasn't had the negative personality disorder or behavior that is supposedly an inevitable part of this, and that's what makes me wonder if they're really right about his condition. The neurologist says his muscles are fine, but the problem is that his brain doesn't communicate with his hands because his brain cells are deteriorating. There is no real way to test for FTD except to biopsy the brain, which of course they don't want to do.

PB: My father died at the age of about eighty-six, and he had a mild form of Alzheimer's that got worse toward the end of his life. He was finally admitted to the hospital where he died. He had some of the symptoms Tom has, and he really wasn't himself anymore. We could communicate but not in a meaningful way. He did become violent with my mother once, so she became afraid of him.

At one point, we had to take the car keys when it was no longer safe for him to drive. I had to physically stop him from getting in the car, and I just said, "Well you know, Dad, you're not in any shape to drive, so we can't let you." He became almost like a little boy and could no longer conduct himself like an adult because things just didn't compute for him.

Annie: That makes so much sense—that he could no longer conduct himself as an adult and became like a little boy.

PB: His sister, my Aunt Jane, was in a nursing home with Alzheimer's disease for about seven years, and she became very dysfunctional. None of this answers your question about whether Tom's diagnosis is correct, but from everything you have said about his thorough workup, they are probably not far off. Doctors would not make a diagnosis like this lightly. At least you know there *is* something wrong with his brain that is causing him to deteriorate, and it's not just a psychological problem. His brain is simply not computing correctly or making connections normally. This is all beyond his control, and the doctors don't think it's reversible.

Annie: Right.

PB: You said he is doing better in terms of his behavior and personality than their diagnosis would suggest, so he may have been helped by the spiritual healer you contacted or by all the medications he is taking. Since you said there's no way to really test him to determine the degree of deterioration he has, you do have to wait it out to see what happens. In any case, according to the doctors, he's not going to get better, and he will probably deteriorate more. My feeling is that they are right, but who knows? I know the uncertainty itself must be hard.

Annie: Yes, it is. So far, he has deteriorated quite quickly in terms of his ability to do things, his interest in activities he used to love, and his ability to relate with me or others as he used to. The doctors were really shocked that within six months he went from holding a demanding job where he was trusted with complex technical assignments to being psychotic and unable to function enough to drive a car or even use a computer. Now he can no longer eat with a fork. In their view, the disease is progressing quickly.

PB: It must be devastating for you to hear what is likely to happen to him and that his condition is terminal.

Annie: I actually felt a little relief when they told me it was terminal, because his life is going to be so difficult. I would rather see him move on to be in the spirit world where he can be whole again than to stay in this limbo.

PB: Then a question for me to ask you is this: If his disease should move along rapidly and he goes relatively soon, can you live with that and be okay?

Annie: Yes. I've always been sort of in charge of taking care of myself. I do have a lot of regrets about things we haven't been able to resolve, so I wonder if we will be together in the spirit world. Have we overcome the things we needed to? I want to leave this life without regrets. I do want that.

I also wonder about what is coming next: What would happen if I got sick? If something happens to me, who would take care of me or Tom? I'm not that emotionally dependent on Tom, but I'm losing my love of life, and I feel like I'm just surviving; just taking care of physical necessities. It's so frustrating that I can't communicate with Tom or have a real relationship with him anymore, and that makes me feel very lonely.

STAYING IN THE PRESENT

PB: Whether we think of it this way or not, life really is a moment-to-moment, hour-to-hour, day-to-day experience. It's because of our vivid imagination and memory that we don't notice that we always cope with life as it comes to us in the moment. There is no way we *can* cope with life in the past or the future, yet you're saying that you are most concerned about missing your relationship as it was in the past and about what might happen in the future.

Focusing on the past or the future can make us feel overwhelmed in the present, but if you spend more time just experiencing this moment, you may see things from a different perspective. You have not changed, but your perception about your life has changed. Your situation requires that you look at each moment in the context of a longer time so you can plan ahead, and you're therefore looking at life more broadly, but you are not really different today than you were before. None of us can live more than one day or even one moment at a time. I say this to you because you have to find a realistic basis for going on so you won't be undone by all that's happening.

Problems are never given to us for the purpose of undoing us, but many in your shoes may ask, "Why me?" Feeling that life is unfair or this shouldn't have happened makes us take on the victim role, and that's exactly what makes us unable to cope. Our better option is to slow down, become more introspective, and observe our lives more closely when life demands much of us. People who are able to do this find new coping skills. They realize they have been living one moment at a time all along but life hasn't demanded that they reflect on it as closely.

Annie: Right.

PB: As you go back into your own history, you'll realize that you've often had some kind of struggle, problem, or challenging situation to deal with. Everyone has that in some way, shape, or form. You coped with all of those challenges, whether they were in relation to Tom, the children, or yourself. You did it moment by moment, and you didn't throw your hands up in despair.

You have had a life of faith, and you still have a life of faith, so you can call on that. Asking yourself where you are in relation to trusting a higher power—that's a large question for you. Is God still there for me? Is God still providing for me and Tom? Is God aware of our situation? Does God still love us? Is God taking care of us? My answer to these questions is, yes, yes, yes, yes, and yes. Life in the past demonstrated that God was always there aiding and guiding. And life in the future will tell you the same thing if you watch for that and see how it is happening right now. Nothing has changed in that sense.

You're having to examine your life and find new reasons to go on, but you can also look back and visit how you successfully faced challenges in the past. For example, how did you cope with relationship problems when Tom was well?

Annie: Well, we could communicate and work on whatever problem we were having. What's difficult now is that I don't know what to do to make anything better between us, and I miss all the good things that were always there.

PB: Of course.

Annie: Many of those good things are now missing, so there is no longer anything to balance out the hard times. Our relationship is really different now.

PB: When Supreme Court Justice Sandra Day O'Connor of Arizona left the Court, she came home to a husband with Alzheimer's disease who thought he was in love with another woman in the nursing home where he was living. In a television interview she talked about how she coped with that situation. It was devastating for her that the person she had loved and been married to for so many years was simply no longer there, even though his body remained alive.

In the end, it's a conscious choice to awaken ourselves to the higher and broader awareness where such an experience can teach us how greatly present God is with us. If we can go more inward, we'll find greater strength within ourselves than we knew we had. Rather than constantly replaying thoughts such as, "I have no one to talk to, I can't cope," or "I don't know what to do," become aware of how you're thinking and do your best to dispel thoughts that are fear-oriented. Sadness and frustration are normal responses to what you're dealing with, so be patient with yourself, but also be as determined and consistent as you can be, because fearful thoughts simply don't serve you.

Annie: Right. I think fear really causes all the havoc. It's hard to deal with all the what-ifs or try to prepare for the future, because I don't know what's going to happen or when.

PB: At its worst, my father's bout with Alzheimer's lasted only about two and a half years before he passed on, and during those two years my mother put everything on hold. When he went into the hospital, she seemed greatly relieved because she was also in her eighties, and there was no way she could cope with caring for him at home any longer.

My wife, Vivien, witnessed her own mother's struggle with dementia. Her mother and father were very close; then they could no longer communicate, and then she was gone. Not long after she went into a care facility, he changed very fast and developed some kind of dementia himself.

I don't think anyone can find an easy explanation for this kind of life event. It just is what it is. It's like watching a weird play and having it do a number on your head. You have to step away from it, become very objective, and find your own life, moment by moment, and day by day.

ACCEPTING HELP

PB: Let the medical system, nursing home, day care, or other service providers cope with the medical side of the problem. As much as you can, turn the physical care over to the professionals, because there comes a time when it's not realistic to think you can deal with it on your own. It may not help you to hear me say all of this because it requires another shift for you, but unless you embrace your reality as opposed to fighting it, it will be doubly difficult.

Annie: The kids keep telling me to get more health aides to come in—to get more assistance— because right now, I'm just going to work, coming home, and taking care of Tom every evening. Then I'm stressed out . . .

PB: Does your insurance cover aides coming in?

Annie: I could probably have more help than I have requested.

PB: Get all the help you can. Vivien works for a company that manages long-term care for people who are ill or disabled, and she connects them with aides and other resources that provide caregivers with help. It makes a big difference, especially when one older person is trying to take care of another. So if part of your story is that you're going to feel guilty if you're not personally taking care of him, let that go. It's just a story.

Annie: Yes, that's exactly it! I ask myself, "Why would I hire somebody when I'm here?" or, "Is he going to feel neglected or think I don't care about him?"

PB: I'll tell you exactly why you need to have help. You're still living, and you may live for many more years, whereas he may go on to the spirit world relatively soon. On a practical level, there are medical and community services available and you have long-term care insurance. See this as God's way of working in your life. All this goodness is God. Just keep remembering that you're going to go on, so you have to find a way to go on happily, positively, and constructively, for *you*. No one is going to do that for you but you. No one.

Annie: Right.

PB: I'm sure your friends are concerned, but they have limited time and energy too, so who is going to help you? Maybe your children, though they also have other commitments. The sooner you become almost clinically objective and take steps to get available help, the sooner you will feel less overwhelmed and he will have the care he really needs. Getting help from service providers doesn't mean you don't care about Tom, but unless you love and care for yourself too, you can't love him. I think you know that.

Annie: Right. And if I go down, I can't take care of him.

PB: Yes. People in your situation sometimes need permission to feel or do a certain thing, and I think you're looking for permission to get the help that's available. You can't quite give yourself permission because you think that if you don't provide the physical care yourself, you're not loving or giving enough. And that's just not true. Be detached enough to let other caregivers take care of Tom as much as possible.

Do you have people around you who can support you on an ongoing basis?

Annie: Well, I joined an Alzheimer's group which includes a lot of people whose loved ones have passed away. They are very helpful in terms of saying to get on with my life, and they are very close friends with each other. They've been the most help to me. Some others don't relate that well to what I'm going through.

PB: Not unless they have the same problem.

Annie: Yes. My boss has an eighty-eight-year-old mother who has Alzheimer's, and we talk a lot. We share lots of stories, and he's very compassionate and sensitive to my situation. Another person in our office had a stroke last year at the age of fifty-five, and we all went through that with him. He recovered quickly but has permanent disability from the stroke and goes through frustrations with that. I can relate to what he goes through. So people in the office are a wonderful support. I also have a women's group that I share with.

No one around me really has an understanding of what's going on in the spirit world though, and that's what I need—a sense that God is in charge, and that this is not some random horrible thing that's happened to us. I need to see it as the kind of thing that sometimes happens to people as part of life and as an opportunity for growth for both of us.

PB: Yes. So my recommendation is to accept and embrace that Tom's life is the way it is. Ensure that he has the care he needs, and do what you need to do to survive—not just physically and practically, but psychologically and emotionally. You have to take good care of yourself. Doing that will be good for both of you, so find the time to relax, to go and have fun, to go to the movies, and to go out to dinner. Be comforted that God is taking care of Tom, and know that everything that is happening is part of a plan. By going through all of this successfully, you are generating very positive karma for yourselves, so the best thing any of us can do in such a situation is to embrace it.

Annie: Well, that helps. Maybe I've been trying to turn the clock back and go back to the way things used to be. I'm trying somehow to make that happen, but I can't. I have been trying to go backward instead of accepting Tom's situation and moving forward. I keep wondering, "What is he thinking? What is he feeling if I hire somebody else or go out and don't take him with me, or whatever? Am I abandoning him?"

PB: In your best-case scenario, what would you think he's thinking?

Annie: On the positive side? I guess that he would want me to be happy.

PB: Yes.

Annie: I guess that's the thing that has kept me wondering. I can't get into his head, so I don't know what he is experiencing. But he doesn't seem to feel embarrassed or neglected. I'm the one projecting that by asking, "Is he thinking that? Is he feeling that?" He just does his thing, hangs out, and seems fine. I'm the one going through all my little mental and emotional issues.

EARTHLY CONTRACTION—
SPIRITUAL EXPANSION

PB: Because of the deterioration of his brain, the higher functions of his mind and even his character and personality are blocked in terms of thoughts, feelings, and behaviors he can experience and express. The neurons in his brain don't connect like they used to, and that's why he is confused. But I have no doubt that he is going out of his body at night into the spirit world and that he is perfectly himself at these times.

His spiritual mind and spiritual body have not been harmed at all but his physical brain is badly damaged, and that's the vehicle he uses to express himself through his physical body. That's not going to get better. Even if the healer you consulted and the treatment he has received are able to help, the damage has probably gone too far for his brain function to come back.

Annie: Right. His brain cells are already damaged.

PB: Yes. So it's better for you to face that squarely and take comfort in knowing that he can still go out of his body to spend time in the spirit world. There, he can express himself perfectly and receive guidance about this whole situation. He can't communicate or function well through his physical body, so you could think of this period of his life as down time for him in this world. He is having more and more enriching experiences in the spirit world and is being prepared to enter that world fully. We can celebrate that when it happens. How a person goes is less important than their state of preparation when they go, and his transition should not be so difficult since he has always been aware of the spirit world.

We might think that people who live a full life and die in their sleep at age ninety-plus are the lucky ones because they get to live a long life and die an easy death; but that's not necessarily so. Perhaps they might have greater spiritual strength or merit if they were to live through the kind of challenges you and Tom are facing. Does this make any sense to you?

Annie: Yes. And I hadn't thought of it that way before. I have been constantly wondering what he's thinking, but you've given me an idea that he may not be thinking very much. He is probably just as he appears and not thinking very deeply at all.

PB: No question about it.

Annie: He's not aware of what people around him are going through, and he's just not connected to the reality of what's happening.

PB: No question about it. So, instead of feeling sorry for him, know that he is spiritually whole in terms of his existence when he goes out of his body. He is continuing to learn and grow on that plane, and this will be to his great credit once he is living completely in the spirit world.

Ultimately, none of us has control over how our life closes. We may think we do, but we don't. Every one of us, whether we are rich, famous, or otherwise, faces an uncertain closure to our physical lives, and the only certain thing is that it's going to happen. The best attitude to take is to embrace whatever happens, because in God's wisdom it is for our highest good. Even if we die a violent death or suffer from cancer, once we step out of the physical body into the spirit world, all the merit of having lived through such a challenge is part of our spirit. Our spirit is actually enlarged because we gain greater compassion and understanding.

Again, while Tom cannot perceive or communicate through his physical body, in spirit he knows very much what's going on. He is aware of you and all you do for him, even though he knows nothing about it in his waking state. When he visits the spirit world, he can communicate with spiritual beings about what you and the children are going through. He can't do anything about it, but he is aware that it's all part of the karmic path for all of you.

Annie: So he can communicate with others in the spirit world, but he can't communicate with us about the situation?

PB: Absolutely. Trying to communicate using his brain is like trying to make a call on a broken telephone. He is fine, but the telephone is broken. I'm not suggesting he is normal mentally except for his ability to communicate. When he is out of his physical body, he has full use of his spiritual mind, but when he is in his physical body, he has extremely limited use of his physical brain.

The great guru, Ramakrishna Paramahansa, a saintly man in India, died of throat cancer, and the pain he experienced during his physical decline was excruciating. He conveyed to his concerned followers that his body was suffering but not "he." He knew that he was not his body, and that he was paying off karma during this life. The payment of karma is the only explanation that is reasonable to me when I think of human suffering. Otherwise, life doesn't make sense. I say this based not only on logic but also because it's the only reality I see as just. I can accept situations like the one you are in because of the concept of karma.

This is a journey for both of you. And from my experience with the spirit world, your husband asked for this. You might ask, "Why would he do that? Why would we, as a couple, ask for this?" It's because we came to earth to grow by undergoing a wide variety of life experiences. In this way, we find our inner strength and find out who we really are. This illness is Tom's roadmap and his destiny. How do we know? Because it is reality, and we can't do anything about it. If you look at it this way, what's happening to both of you is inevitable.

You married Tom, and he married you. You have children in common, and you have shared many life experiences. He'll go on ahead of you, and that's a part of the plan, too. The man you know will be waiting for you in the spirit world, and you can resume your relationship with him then. Instead of resisting reality and having your own idea of how things should go, embrace everything that *is*. If you can do this, you'll find that much of the pain will subside and you can better adjust. Does this help?

Annie: Yes; very much so.

PB: What are you feeling now? Go inside and ask yourself what you're feeling as we're talking about your situation.

Annie: I guess I'm trying to make the internal shift from worrying about what's going to happen, about where Tom is, and about what he is thinking to feeling that on some level everything's okay. Whatever he is going through, that's his journey. I can support him, but I'm not going to be able to communicate with him the way I used to.

PB: Yes.

LIVING WELL
AS INDIVIDUALS

PB: In the larger, eternal scheme of things, you can view what is happening to you and Tom not only as adversity, but as opportunity. What does this mean? Well, we've mentioned the concept of karma, and we could also look at the possibility that this situation will help you discover deeper aspects of yourself. Sometimes husbands and wives become so codependent that their lives overlap to the point that they lose themselves as individuals.

Annie: Yes.

PB: Now is the time to look at your own life and the things you want to accomplish—not in a self-centered or egotistical way but by using common sense. What do you want to experience in life that you've not yet experienced? For example, suppose you love live theater, movies, or art. Give yourself permission to go and experience what you enjoy, and don't deprive yourself of such things. It's good for both you and Tom if you do things that are restorative for you, because you'll feel more positive when you're with him, and he'll pick up on that energy. Whether Tom remains chronically disabled for a long time or moves on into the spirit world soon, now is the time to begin thinking about what you can do to fulfill your own life.

Vivien and I have overlapping lives in many ways, and we communicate a lot, especially about our children and grandchildren, but since the age of sixty, we have intentionally become more independent of each other so we can each fulfill our own inner needs. We go on some vacations together and some separately. For example, I encouraged her to go to see her family alone because I knew she'd come back and tell me about her experiences. I could share them with her that way, and it was great that she could be with her siblings without me.

Annie: She could be free to interact the way she wants to with her family.

PB: And she experiences a greater portion of herself. It can be the same for me when she's not here. We do some things separately for very positive reasons. If couples have a strong bond of love between them, that's not going to go away if they have a degree of independence. And if couples are too codependent, one may die shortly after the other.

Annie: Yes.

PB: A survivor who has a number of personal interests to help them carry on may live for many more years.

Annie: Right. I can definitely visualize that very easily. I just have to give myself permission to stop focusing all my attention on Tom and his situation.

PB: Yes. And you will. You're a very intelligent woman. You articulate very well, and what I'm most impressed by is your ability to be objective. I really admire that, and it will serve you well in this situation. Sometimes we have to be very objective to make decisions that ensure our own welfare as well as that of our loved one.

Sandra Day O'Connor spoke very objectively about what happened to her husband. Why? As a judge, she had to look at facts, information, and stories with detachment, so she was able to look at her husband's situation the same way. You could see that she was in great pain at the loss of what they had, but she was not going to fool herself or pretend it was otherwise, so she dropped the story of their former relationship. She will probably resume it when they are both in the spirit world, but for now she is going on independently to be productive in her own right. What other choice does she have?

Annie: It's hard to accept that you can't really know the other person's journey.

PB: Well, what if the shoe were on the other foot? What would you want Tom to do? You would want him to take the best care of you he could, but if he didn't have the coping skills, or if he had to hold down a job, you would not want him to give up his whole life because your life had changed. You would also want him to take advantage of the help available through insurance and community resources.

Annie: That's true. You can only do the best you can do. I know he would do the best he could, and I'm sure, on some level, he knows I'm doing the best I can.

PB: I know it hurts you to see him go through having food on his face and having to wear a diaper, because you want to protect his dignity, but remember that those are external, superficial, and temporary conditions. It's how things are, so the most important thing is to ensure that he has the best care possible. Doing that is the best way to protect his dignity right now.

Annie: Yes.

THE BOOK OF LIFE

PB: I imagine the logical part of your mind is still trying to make sense of all that is happening to you and Tom, but some things just don't compute. Life has so many mysteries that I have stopped asking some of the questions I used to ask. I just know there is a plan; so no matter what happens, I embrace it. Even if I don't know the details, I believe I signed up for whatever happens in my life.

It took me a number of years to get to this point, but it happened when I finally realized I was creating a lot of pain for myself by fighting reality. For example, because I'm a medium, I never have a time when I'm not "on" because, at least in my experience, I have to stay aligned with spirit through prayer and meditation in order to bring the best to people when they come to me. Because people are always waiting for a reading, I'm never free from that responsibility, and part of me would like to be. I finally embraced all of this as my reality and said, "Father, thank you for trusting me with work that is often such an important part of people's lives. Whatever you send my way, I embrace it. I'm not going to fight it anymore, and I'm not going to think it should be otherwise." When I could say that and mean it, things shifted for me, and I began to feel greater peace.

Annie: That's just how it is.

PB: Yes. I'm very fortunate if I look at my life from the standpoint of having the great opportunity and blessing of helping people help themselves. When I stopped thinking it should be otherwise and dropped my story that I shouldn't have to carry the weight of this responsibility, I felt much better.

Annie: That makes a lot of sense.

PB: Well, that's because you can't fight reality. Any time you do, you lose. I think of reality as God, because nothing can happen outside of God. So instead of fighting reality, I embrace it.

I tell myself and people I work with, "Whatever is bothering you and whatever you don't want to face, turn around and walk toward it. Walk right into it, even if it's very painful and seems impossible to do, because in doing that you'll knock the problem down to size and put it in the right perspective." When we do that, the situation will change. Things will get better, and the problem will either go away or at least be easier to live with. We will not have the same degree of discomfort we had before.

Annie: I just wrote that down: "Knock it down to size and put it in the right perspective."

PB: Well, the *Book of Revelations* refers to the *Book of Life*. What is the *Book of Life*? Like any book, life unfolds chapter by chapter. Chapter 1 of our lives is different from Chapter 50, and each chapter is an episode that includes an opportunity to learn and grow. Okay, you're at this chapter now, and it may be very different from the previous one and the one that follows. Each chapter is a unique unit, and we need to learn everything we can from each one. So when I look at what's happening in my life, I ask what I'm supposed to learn from it.

In having this conversation, we are not really talking about Tom's situation but your own. You can't live his life, so we're talking about your life. I think you get that.

Annie: Right.

PB: Then you can ask, "What is this experience with Tom teaching me about me? What is it that this chapter of my life is telling me to look at, to learn, to wake up to, or to correct?" When you begin to look at your life from this perspective, it's much easier to live out each chapter.

Annie: Yes. I have been feeling as though I'm entering another part of my life, and I have had no idea where I am right now. This is such a different ball park. In the past, I learned how to use a lot of tools to improve my marriage, but they just don't apply to our relationship now. I know I'm in a different chapter of my life, but I have been having a lot of trouble getting focused on how to make it rich, purposeful, and good.

PB: Yes, those are beautiful words—"rich, purposeful, and good." Have you found yourself able to become more philosophical about what is going on?

Annie: I'm beginning to. I've been dragged down with physical work and worry, including anxiety about how to work things out. But I'm aware that this is the time to become more internally focused. I know it's detrimental to keep focusing on physical realities I can't control. My mind just needs to be more focused on living in the present and preparing for the future rather than longing for the past.

PB: Well, this is what destiny handed you, and God never hands us these kinds of things for our undoing. We can always use them as a stepping stone to go higher.

Annie: Right. I've always struggled with taking care of my own health, and Tom's condition just puts that issue right in my lap. If I don't take care of me, I can't go on taking care of him.

PB: Well, if you don't take care of yourself, you'll be in bed right beside him, figuratively speaking.

Annie: I can't wait too long to start taking care of myself.

PB: No, you can't.

Annie: And if I go downhill, there's nobody to take care of me, so my health needs to be a priority. It's what I've needed all along, even when Tom was well, to focus on taking better care of my health, and I've never been good at that.

PB: Well, you raised two children, worked on your relationship with your husband, held a job, and spent a lot of time taking care of other people and situations. Now is the time to devote more energy to you, even as you look out for Tom's welfare.

Annie: Right. I just need to take advantage of the opportunity to have the aides help out more and focus on my own health and mental state. I want to leave this earth feeling grateful and full of life, not feeling miserable.

PB: Well your voice has a very "up" vibration now. And from the beginning of our conversation, I haven't detected any self-pity.

Annie: I don't feel sorry for myself. I'm just struggling to get on top of things and see a positive vision of how to make this a rich and good experience. I guess my constant worry has been about what he is going through and what I should be doing, plus the concern that I'm letting him down somehow. I'm recently realizing that I don't smile much anymore, so I know I'm losing my joy. I just want my life back.

PB: Your zest for living?

Annie: Right. I don't want to lose that.

A DIFFERENT
RELATIONSHIP

PB: You can model yourself in the image of a nurse practitioner or psychiatric nurse in your relationship with Tom, and that could serve you both well. You're no longer able to function in the role of wife, even if you do the best you can, because he can't reciprocate at that level. And for the most part, that's not what he needs from you anymore, because he can no longer function in his role as a husband. What he can relate to is to someone who is objective about his situation who helps him get his meds on time, get to the day care center on time, eat properly, and stay clean. The more you can see yourself in that role, the easier it will be for both of you.

Annie: That's tremendously helpful, because that's what I've been struggling with: "How can I be a wife when I can't communicate with my husband, and he seems more like a son to me?" Our life just doesn't work the way it used to, and the tools I used to build our relationship don't work because his brain isn't there anymore. If I function more like a caring, compassionate nurse who takes care of his needs, that will work better.

I also like the idea that he can actually be in the spirit world in his dreams or when he is out of his body during sleep and have communication with spirit beings about everything. He can interact at a deep level and receive rich spiritual food, so I don't have to worry about that part of his life. That's very reassuring to me, because I don't want him to feel alone or neglected. The idea that spiritual beings are taking care of him and preparing him for his transition—that he has a rich spiritual life—is very comforting to me.

PB: He does have that, though people, including those in the medical field, don't understand this. Because I'm clairvoyant and clairaudient, I know without a doubt, moment to moment and day by day, that the other world exists, and that gives me a great advantage in bringing that information to those who are open to it.

Tom is not really suffering in spirit, though profound limitations have come upon his body. His soul is free. If you take the view that this is just how he decided to go to the other side, you will experience less grief about it. It's natural to mourn what has been lost in terms of your relationship, but Tom is not even aware of that loss, so he is not suffering as much as you are.

At my funeral I don't want anyone crying. I want people to be happy—partying, blowing horns and whistles, and dancing—because they can say to themselves, "Philip has moved on to the other world. How lucky he is to be in a better place beyond this earth plane!"

As I wrote in one of my books, I was in Dallas many years ago staying with someone who was providing pastoral support to hospice patients admitted to the hospital. He must have told the hospital to call me if he wasn't available, because the hospital called and asked me to visit a dying man who needed a minister. I was with another friend who knew Dallas, so we jumped in his car and sped to the hospital.

I hurried to the third floor, expecting to see someone take his last breath, but the man I came to visit was sitting up in bed. His wife was sitting on the foot of his bed, leaning on the wall, sound asleep and looking totally exhausted. I said to the hospice patient, "They told me you were dying," and he replied, "I thought I was, but I'm not now!" I asked him what was happening, and he said, "Well, last night my wife was sitting by my bed right where you are now, and suddenly I felt myself rising up toward the ceiling. I said, 'Hold my hand! Hold my hand; I'm dying!' And I went all the way up to the ceiling. I looked down at my body and I could see that my wife was holding my hand. Then I came back down and into my body again."

I said, "Sir, you have had an out-of-body experience. This is the same thing that happens when we die, but we just don't come back into the body as you did this time. If you had actually died, you would have gone on, but in this case, it was not your time to go. You have experienced how people make their transition into the spirit world and what death is like. The spirit doesn't die; only the body, and now you have this wonderful insight. You have been allowed to have it so that when you die it will be much easier for you. You now know exactly what to expect."

My explanation relieved him a lot. He stopped being agitated and was very much at peace. We talked for about an hour longer, and he was smiling and laughing much of that time. His wife never woke up! She must have been taking care of him to the point of exhaustion, and she probably needed help more than he did.

This story serves well to say to you, "Take care of yourself. Tom will be all right. Everything is in divine order, and God is holding Tom's hand and taking care of him." He has also surrounded you both with angels and other spirit beings to help you.

Annie: Yes. I can believe we're getting that kind of help, and it's much better than the way I have been looking at things. One example is that we took out a long-term care insurance policy for Tom before he became ill. We couldn't even get a policy for me because my health wasn't good, but he was in perfect health, so we decided to get one for him, even though we couldn't afford it. When we found out about his condition, we both thought it was more than a coincidence that we had purchased the insurance. We asked ourselves, "How could it be that we decided to get long-term care insurance and then had it work out so well for us?" It has made all the difference. Now Tom can be taken care of. Also, whether they're correct or not, the doctors gave Tom the diagnosis of being terminally ill, and that helped us get disability right away. Many people struggle for years to get disability, but it was no problem for us. So we've been blessed. I've been able to keep a sense of gratitude that Tom is very well taken care of and seems quite happy. I can see that I'm the one who struggles.

PB: Yes, of course. Again, for your sake, it's good that you can be objective instead of taking the attitude that you're a victim. If you accept everything that's happening as your destiny and as an opportunity to pay off karma and move forward on your path, you will have greater confidence in your ability to get through this.

Annie: I know I'll be better off if I can focus on the good fortune we've had with the care we're getting. I just need to make the best decisions I know how to make and keep on going. The issue for me now is to get joy back and find my spiritual center instead of focusing on all the problems. They get my attention because they demand it, but if I can get more aides to help and stop feeling guilty about going out alone or with other people, maybe I can get my life back.

PB: Well, as we've said, if your life becomes so intertwined with the downside of Tom's life that you go down, too, that's no good for either one of you.

Annie: Yes. I am very aware of that, and it's actually the main reason I called you. I just feel like I can't go down, because then I'm no good to anybody—myself, Tom, or the kids. I want to be a strong, joyful spiritual center for all of them, and I don't want the kids to be always worrying about me. They're beginning to wonder if they're going to have to take care of me too because they see me falling apart under the stress of taking care of him. They're already telling me to get more help. I guess it's finally getting through to me that I can gratefully accept all the help I can get, and I don't need to feel guilty.

PB: No, you do not.

Annie: When I think like that, my situation feels much lighter. I can say, "Let's just deal with the physical part," knowing that all of this has some kind of eternal meaning and value. Going through this makes me recognize that my own years are limited, and I really want to do the most I can with the time I have left. I haven't been able to make that happen before now, but this conversation will help. I especially appreciate your advice to take on the role of being more like a nurse, because that's what Tom needs now. I like that idea much better than feeling like I have to be like a mother, and that's what I have been feeling. I don't *want* to be Tom's mother! But the idea of being his nurse until we reconnect later in the spirit world feels better and makes more sense.

CHANGING
NEEDS

PB: When my Aunt Jane had Alzheimer's, each time I visited her she had deteriorated more, and finally she was in a nursing home, bedridden and curled up in a ball. She was my favorite aunt, but at some point, she couldn't remember who I was. I recall that she had a strong body odor because of incontinence, and this is something she would never have allowed when she was well. I knew her brain could no longer detect or interpret the odor around her and that she couldn't function normally, so I felt only compassion for her.

Annie: Right. Tom doesn't notice if he has food all over his face or if his diaper is dirty or wet.

I'll ask him to wash his face, but he doesn't even see what I'm talking about, and he doesn't smell anything when his diaper needs changing. All those senses are gone or don't mean anything to him.

PB: Yes. So in that sense, he is more like an infant, and that's how it is.

Annie: Right. I've also noticed that he seems most comfortable when he is receiving care from people other than me or one of the children. At the day care center he seems to feel like everybody is in the same boat and he's no different from anyone else, but at home he's different from us and from who he was before so it's harder. The truth is that I don't know if he is even aware of the difference, so I may just be projecting, but I know he seems comfortable receiving help at the day care center.

PB: Well, we all feel comfortable with people who are most like us, however we are.

Annie: Right. I think he loves us, but he seems to be comfortable and more at ease just being able to relax and do whatever everybody else is doing at the day care center. At home he is constantly confronted with all the things he can't do—all the things he used to do and can't anymore. I don't know how much I'm projecting, but it seems that way to me.

PB: If you continue to yearn, even subconsciously, for a normal relationship where you exchange feedback as equal partners, energetically that's going to be a burden for both of you, because it's not a possibility.

Annie: Yes, that's the problem. I want to go back to where I could connect with him, and I just have to let that go. It isn't going to happen again in this life.

PB: No, it's not. In terms of helping him, the less you focus on what was, the better it is for both of you.

Annie: I can see that if I carry that expectation, it would put a burden on him that he can't carry and cause me to feel constantly frustrated.

PB: Yes. He might not be consciously aware of it, but if you harbor an expectation that he can't meet, he will feel it on some level. Your energy around that expectation will still be there to draw upon his, and you don't want to do that. I know it's not easy. It's hard to step into the role of being an objective nurse when you've been in a loving, intimate relationship as Tom's wife. But on the other hand, it's even harder to cling to the role of being his wife when that's no longer possible. Things are different now, so it will be easier if you can adjust and act accordingly. I do know it's not easy.

Sometimes, when an emergency happens, I become a different person. I literally become very detached, in a positive way, and I'm able to take charge without any sense of panic. I've gotten to the point that even if I drop a glass in the kitchen and it breaks on the floor, I don't get upset. I just watch it drop, watch it break, and sweep it up. I have learned how to just observe the "play" of my life, including things that would have caused me frustration, worry, or fear in the past. Doing this brings forward the divinity that's in me and in all of us and allows me to embrace the reality of my situation in a larger sphere, which I call love. It's all love. It's all God—everything that's happening.

This goes back again to the question we've been discussing, "How do I love myself?" You have to consciously love yourself holistically, in detail, and that means loving your life as it is *now*, not as it was or as you want it to be. Just remember that you and Tom can resume your married life as equal partners in the spirit world.

Annie: Right.

PB: Another understanding that helps me is that what I give out is what I will get back. If you're giving out positive and loving energy toward Tom and maintaining a constructive attitude by putting all that's happening in a larger context, you're going to get that positive energy back. Doing that consciously is what self-mastery is all about. You may not be able to do this all the time, but move in that direction as much as you can. I recently read the words, "Show me a hero, and I'll show you a place of great suffering."

When I face adversity, instead of responding with worry or fear, I consciously send positive energy toward it and try to stay objective about it. Whenever I do that, I find positive results and a positive solution, so I know from experience that maintaining objectivity definitely works. For any of us, and especially for you at this time, being as objective as possible will lead you toward self-mastery.

Annie: That sounds right.

IDEAS TO GROW ON

PB: Of all the ideas we've discussed, what is of the greatest value to you?

Annie: Well, there's more than one idea that has great value for me. What really stands out, though, is the idea that Tom's spiritual needs are being met through his out-of-body interaction with God and the various spirit guides that are with him. I don't have to worry about what he's feeling or receiving spiritually because he has a source that is meeting those needs. That gives me permission not to try to meet needs that I can't meet right now. I am also comforted by the idea that what we are going through, in terms of karma, can be valuable and positive for our growth and our eternal future.

The suggestion to become more objective and take the position of a nurse is very valuable because I have been asking myself, "How should I, as Tom's wife, respond to this situation?" I'm realizing through this conversation that I can't expect myself to relate, to be in the role of Tom's wife. The reality is that we're not able to relate to each other that way anymore, but we're so connected that it's hard to stand back and be objective about that. I just haven't been able to find how to navigate that problem, but the idea of being more objective and relating like a compassionate nurse to Tom's condition really helps.

He just came in . . . .

PB: I heard him, and he sounded very normal to me. I heard him ask about dinner.

Annie: Yes, that's it! It's always, "When's my dinner?" not, "Hello, how are you?" But yes, he's very normal in terms of our everyday routine, and I can see he's not suffering unduly. If I'm able to move on and become more joyful myself, I think that will definitely benefit everybody.

PB: Yes, absolutely, because you are the center. That part may not be so different from how it was when Tom was well.

Annie: Yes.

PB: And so that reality is just larger.

Annie: Right. That's not so new to me. I just haven't been able to figure out the part about how we could still be husband and wife the way we used to be or how to continue working on our relationship. Now I think the way to work on it is to let God hold it and move forward more on my own. Now I feel I have permission to focus more on what I need and what I want to work on for myself as long as I make sure he is being properly cared for. That takes a lot of the heaviness away.

PB: It puts things in a different perspective when you have a direction for what to do and greater hope for the future.

Annie: Right.

PB: That's the word I often find missing in situations like this: hope.

Annie: Yes.

PB: Actually, finding hope is part of self-mastery. Hope comes from within you as you put everything into perspective by embracing reality just as it is and not fighting it. Then the energy comes to help you go on.

Annie: Right, because we will all pass away . . .

PB: Well exactly! Only all of us.

Annie: It's natural, but most of us don't really think that through.

PB: No. Sometimes I say to an audience I'm addressing, "You know, I have yet to meet a man or woman who isn't going to die." This shifts everything into a flat-out reality that no one can argue with. In any case, it's a good lead-in to talking about what happens when we die and about what comes next. I can say, "So, here I am to tell you more about that."

Annie: Yes, it was just conceptual to me before, but now that I've started dealing with the reality of the dying process, it's another story.

PB: Yes.

Unless you have questions, I want to say in conclusion that we've covered a lot of ground, and it's unlikely that you could incorporate everything we've said during this span of time.

You may not agree with all I've said, and you may find some parts of our discussion more valuable than others, but you used the word "process" more than once, and that's exactly what you're going through. As you go back over this conversation and review experiences you've had with the Alzheimer's group and others, God will continue to show you the way. There will be little and larger lights that will illuminate your path and show you what's next, what's next, and what's next after that.

Just stay cradled in faith and hope that those who work with you in spirit are very much embracing you and Tom individually and together, and they're helping to point the way for you to go. They're helping to give information and bring about situations as they probably did when you decided to purchase your long-term care insurance. They're there to comfort you and usher you on. They *are* there. And they are part and parcel of everything you and Tom are going through. So if you wake up in the middle of the night and feel lonely, desperate, sad, or grieved, just climb into the arms of a loving spiritual friend. Visualize them there, and they *will* be there. They will help you. They'll help ease the pain, and they'll bring in energies to lift you up and help you carry on.

I live that way all the time. Without the friendship of those who work with me in spirit regarding this work, I would have given up long ago, but I'm aware that they are always there. They'll sometimes wake me up at 3:00 or 4:00 in the morning to bring in information or comfort. Because I'm a medium, I can see them standing there and hear them speak, so their companionship is a living reality for me. You may not see or hear them as I do, but those loving beings specifically assigned to guide you *are* really there. The spirit world *is* helping! We're already living in spirit, and the only difference is that we are still attached to our bodies. Many don't realize this, but it's true.

Do you have any questions you want to ask?

Annie: No, I have a lot to think about, and I'm very grateful for that.

PB: Okay. May I close with a prayer then?

Annie: Yes, please.

CLOSING PRAYER: *Beloved Father, I always start with you and come back to you, and when I think of you, I think of unconditional love. In that unconditional love there is provision for every circumstance—good, bad, or otherwise. You are irrefutably bound up in our destiny* *because you live in us, and while the exterior part of us may be negatively affected due to age or ill health, you are always there within us. And so, you are guiding Annie and Tom through their eternal, divine minds. You are showing them the way day by day, light by light, and situation by situation. You are ushering them individually and together through this chapter of their lives.*

Each of us comes into this life experience and goes out of it as an individual, and all the things we experience from the time we come in to the time we go out are for our edification and learning. May this chapter of Annie's life experience help her to grow in patience and love toward herself and others, becoming a much richer and wiser person spiritually than she could have been if Tom had not become ill. May her experience enlarge her soul so that she can have increased compassion for all people. Help her to experience in heart and mind and demonstrate in action that she loves herself and others unconditionally.

Most of all, may Annie learn that the grand, grand prize of life is already present—you in us and us in you. There's no place to go and nothing to do but to go inside and find your eternal, burning, brilliant light always there. As we turn inward and find you waiting there, we experience the eternal comfort and love that we have been longing for. And this light, this presence of yourself, has not gone out and will not go out in Tom or in any of us. It is that guiding principle, that guiding light, that unconditional love that ever steers our lives toward the right outcomes.

Thank you for this time with Annie. Thank you for the wisdom, understanding, and communication we could share. I ask that you support Annie and her family in every way and bless them abundantly through this experience. I pray all of this in the universal Christ Spirit. Amen.

Annie: *Amen.*

PB: I've recorded our conversation on two CDs, and I'd be more than happy to send them to you, if you would like that.

Annie: Yes, I would appreciate that.

PB: Well, listening again to what *you* had to say allows you to revisit your own realizations and maintain a positive perspective for yourself. God bless you.

ANNIE'S LETTER

Dear Philip,

I was so inspired when I learned you would be using material from our conversation for this publication, and I know it will help many people who are caring for a loved one who has dementia.

Tom continues to decline gradually, and he recently spent five days in the hospital after suddenly collapsing while trying to get dressed. When we took him to urgent care, it turned out that he had extremely low blood pressure, was very dehydrated, and had a urinary tract infection. The doctors were able to stabilize him and send him home with antibiotics, and he has since been doing okay. He is more impatient and demanding now.

However, since my conversation with you, *I'm* doing better, and that makes a big difference to all of us. I'm better at accepting the reality of what's happening, and I continue to work on adjusting my expectations, which helps a lot. I want and need a husband, but Tom can't be that for me anymore, and the more I accept that the less hurt and disappointment I feel. I'm still in the early stages of being able to emotionally separate myself from Tom's inability to relate to me as he used to, but my mindset is gradually shifting. I have my memories, and I know that after he passes over, Tom will be himself again. I was especially comforted when you said he is being nurtured and educated in the spirit world while he is sleeping at night. Remembering that helps me so much.

My conversation with you has also helped me to realize that I need to focus on my own life and live it very positively, so I don't decline along with Tom. I have been able to get more help in caring for Tom, and that gives me more time to replenish myself so I can be more patient and loving when I'm with him. I have found that if I talk about the things he loves that are important to him, like the children's stories he wrote and the time when he taught Sunday School, he is able to be more connected, present, and happy.

Sharing memories of the kids growing up gives us both joy. When I expect Tom to connect to what we are doing now he is very disinterested, which is hurtful and sad for me, so I am learning to shift my expectations and focus on positive things we can share from the past. Doing this helps us both.

I am so grateful to have long-term health insurance for Tom. We got it right before he turned fifty when the rates were going to jump up. It was so hard to pay for, but it has made such a difference in our ability to cope with his illness. The cost of caring for a loved one struck with this kind of condition is so high, and we are lucky that we can be reimbursed for having aides come into our home to help. I could never have afforded this kind of help without the insurance we have.

Last week we got Tom an adjustable bed! He had been sleeping in a recliner for a year because he is uncomfortable lying down flat on a regular bed, but we couldn't afford to buy an adjustable bed because they are very expensive. I finally called my regular health insurance company, and they said that with a doctor's prescription they would cover one hundred percent of the costs for renting an adjustable hospital bed for as long as Tom needs it. He is so happy with his new bed!

He can't figure out the remote control enough to adjust the bed by himself, so we just keep it set in a position that is comfortable for him. I'm continuing to learn that there are resources out there if I ask.

Our son and his family have moved several states away, and our daughter has moved into an apartment with some friends, so it is much quieter around our home now. This is another adjustment for me, and I will really need to focus on getting out more now that the kids aren't around to talk to. I am also looking forward to having more time to read and meditate.

I can't express how grateful I am for my conversation with you, including the insight I gained about how to relate to Tom, your encouragement to keep developing my own life, and your advice to ask for help when I need it. We all have to play out the hand we are dealt in life, and I now feel I have many of the tools I need to see us through Tom's illness.

Thank you, Philip!

With love,
Annie

AFTERWORD

L ife is difficult enough without having to deal
with an illness that incapacitates or leads to
the death of a loved one, especially when that
person is our lifelong mate. I greatly admire
Annie's objective approach to seeking answers
and applying them to her difficult situation
without being undone. All her wifely and moth-
erly instincts came to her aid when the reality
of her husband's illness came rushing into her
awareness, foreshadowing his early death. As a
prospective survivor with perhaps many years
ahead of her, she asked the understandable question, "What is going to happen to me?"

We can all relate. It is not a selfish question but a necessary one. Countless numbers of
spouses who remain on earth after the departure
of a partner ask the same or a similar question:

"What now? What about me?" Being with others in a similar situation can be most helpful in answering that question, and I was pleased to learn that Annie had availed herself of such support.

I wanted to allay Annie's fears and help her give voice to what was in her heart and mind. While I know that she has her own religious and spiritual convictions, I also wanted to put the events surrounding her husband's pressing and serious illness into the largest possible perspective, and this includes an understanding of eternal existence. As we continued our conversation, I could sense Annie's growing self-awareness. She expressed herself with greater ease and peace, whether she was talking about practical or spiritual issues. She recognized truth for herself in the spiritual realities we discussed.

Even if our bodies and minds are severely impaired, we remain eternal beings who have an unbreakable connection with the spirit world. Most people on earth are unaware of this simply because our eternal spiritual nature is not well understood. If it were, humanity would have greater peace in the face of chronic, disabling, and life-threatening illness. We would know that a dear child, husband, wife, mother, or father, is being attended by a circle of spiritual beings who aid them at every turn. These expert and tender beings guide them out of their bodies regularly to visit in the spirit world, helping them to live fully and freely in spirit, even as they lose the ability to do so on earth.

As a child, I consciously left my body at night and entered the spirit world to study with spiritual masters who guided me for many years, and I know this experience is not unique to me. I shared my out-of-body experience with Annie and encouraged her to imagine that her husband was being guided in a similar way, explaining that he is fully aware and well during these spiritual excursions. Since Annie already believes in the afterlife, this idea resonated with her, and it brought the peace of mind that she longed for.

Because of her sincerity and integrity, I have no doubt that Annie will do well as the months and years unfold. As she continues to grow on her own earthly journey through life, she is likely to do herself and her husband a great service by preparing well for their eternal life together at the time when she makes her own transition into the light.

May all who grieve for the loss of a loved one come to realize the full reality of life on earth and in the spirit world—that death does not end life but gives us the chance to live a greater life, unhindered by illness, disability, or lack of spiritual understanding. At the death of the physical body, especially if we are well prepared through our life experience, we enter eternal life to quickly be filled to the brim with the answers to all of our questions, only to be inspired to ask new questions with answers that lead to still greater understanding. We continue on an endless spiritual journey; and we find a larger life of ultimate joy and peace.

—*Philip Burley*

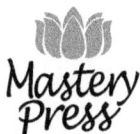

Mastery Press

Phoenix, Arizona

For general inquiries send an email to
PB@PhilipBurley.com, or write to:

Adventures in Mastery, LLC (AIM)
P.O. Box 43548
Phoenix, AZ 85080

For more information about Philip Burley
and the work of
Adventures in Mastery, LLC,
please visit this website:
www.PhilipBurley.com

9 781883 389222